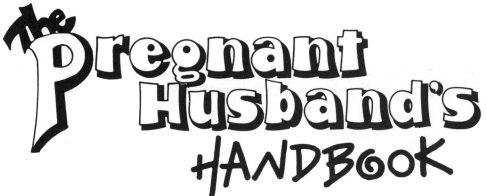

The Pregnant Husband's HANDBOOK

By Jeff Justice

Illustrated by Clark Taylor

Published by Strawberry Patch, Atlanta, Georgia

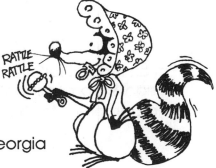

RATTLE RATTLE

Published by: Strawberry Patch
            P.O. Box 52404
            Atlanta, Georgia 30355

Editor: Diane Pfeifer
Design & Composition: Paula Chance, Peachtree Type & Design
Photography: Matthew FitzRandolph

I dedicate this book to my good-natured wife, Diane, and comic daughter, Jennica Snow, without whom this book would not have been possible; and to Sam and Virginia Justice, without whom I would not have been possible; and to God, for giving us all a sense of humor.

Foreword

Pregnant women are very sensitive creatures. Unfortunately, they constantly confront their husbands with questions that can't possibly be answered truthfully without paying a lot of alimony. Having recently fielded these questions myself, I decided to share the appropriate responses to help guide future fathers. Just for fun, I've supplied the right answer along with two painfully incorrect replies. Check your choices in the back of the book to see if you are the perfect "Pregnant Husband".

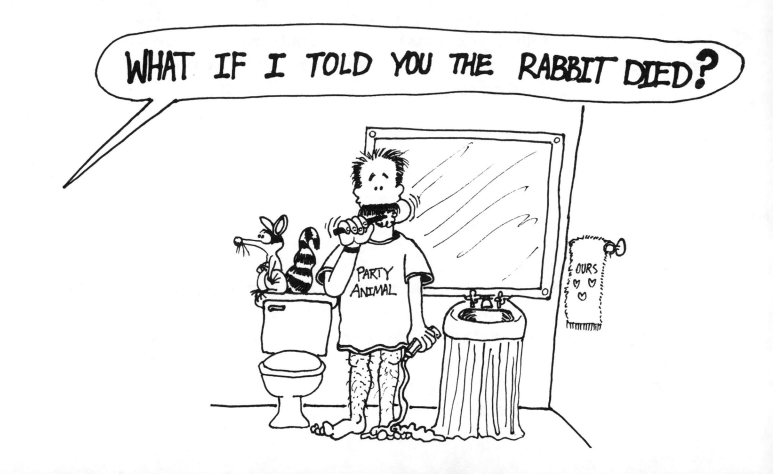

1.

A. I'll start the barbecue.

B. What wine goes with that?

C. Those are the most wonderful words
I've heard since you said, "I do".

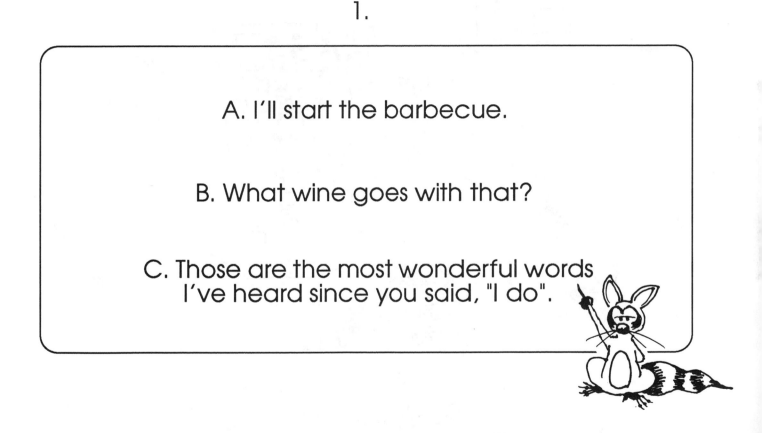

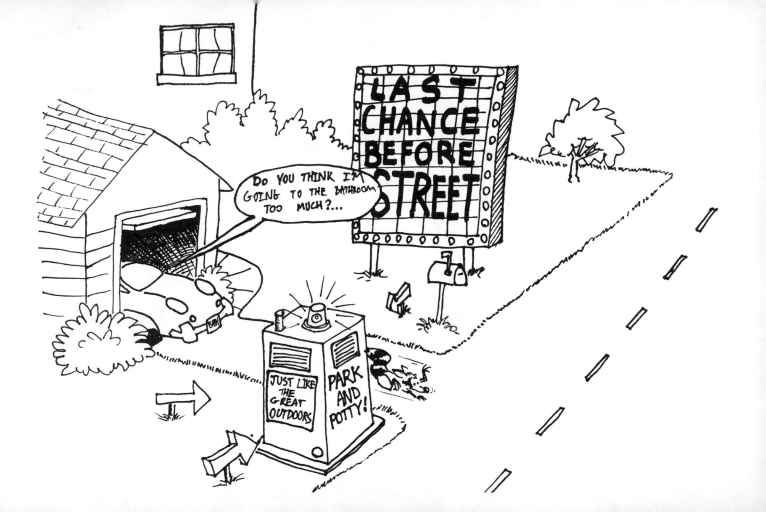

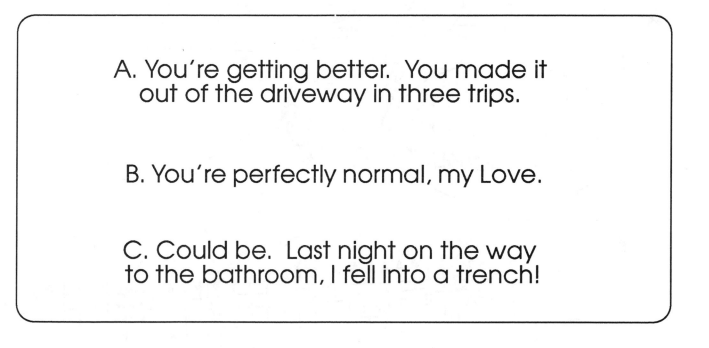

A. You're getting better. You made it out of the driveway in three trips.

B. You're perfectly normal, my Love.

C. Could be. Last night on the way to the bathroom, I fell into a trench!

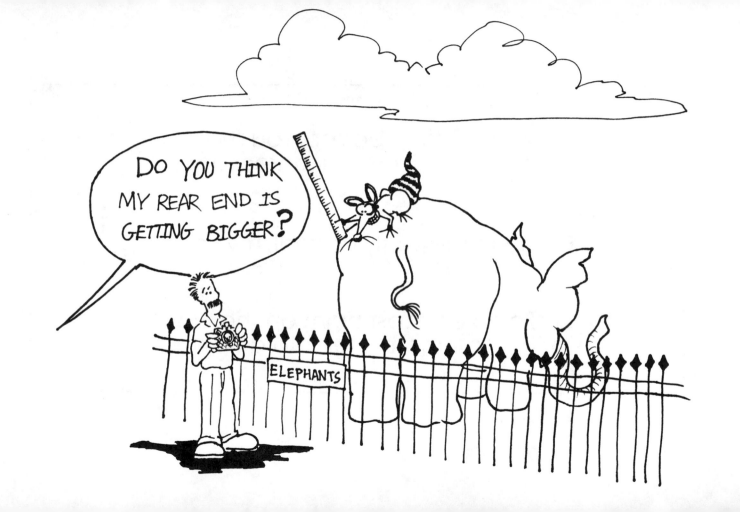

A. No, Baby, sexier!

B. You're just paranoid because that cop made you wear that "extra-wide load" sign.

C. No, even if your jeans do say "U-Haul".

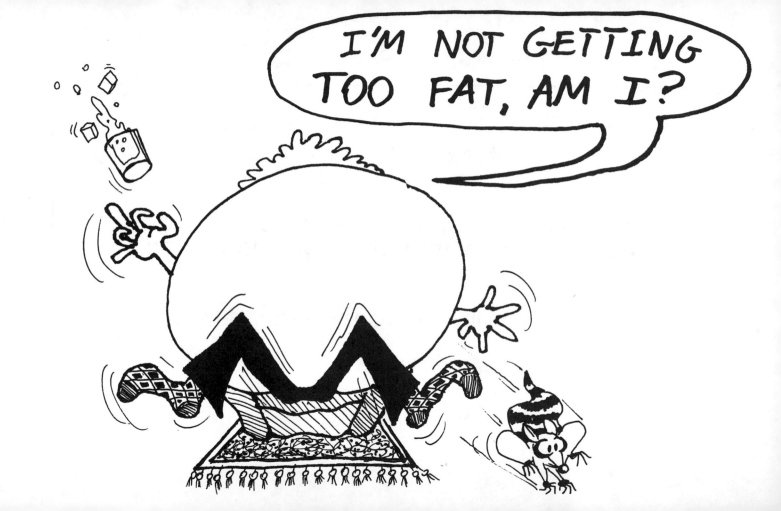

4.

A. Hey, personally I love having our own zip code!

B. I've never seen you look lovelier.

C. No, Cuddles, we needed a bigger house anyway.

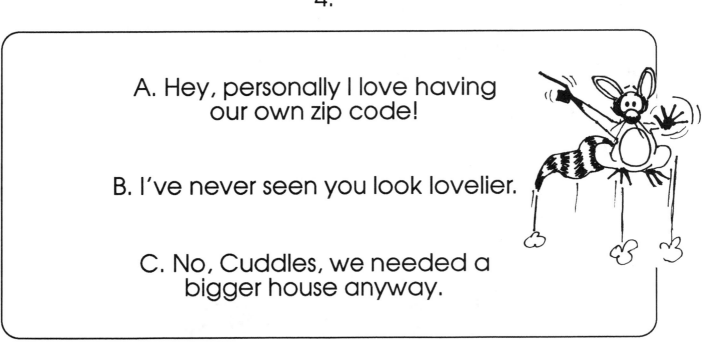

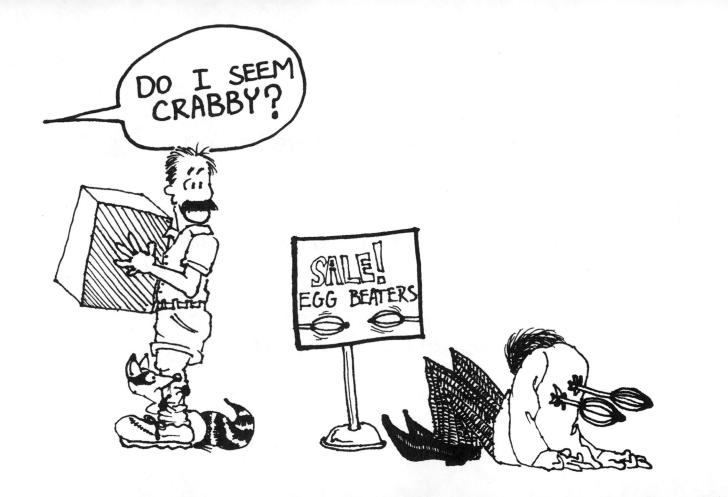

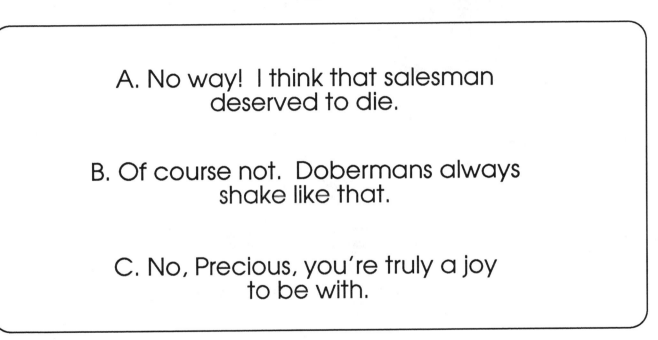

A. No way! I think that salesman
deserved to die.

B. Of course not. Dobermans always
shake like that.

C. No, Precious, you're truly a joy
to be with.

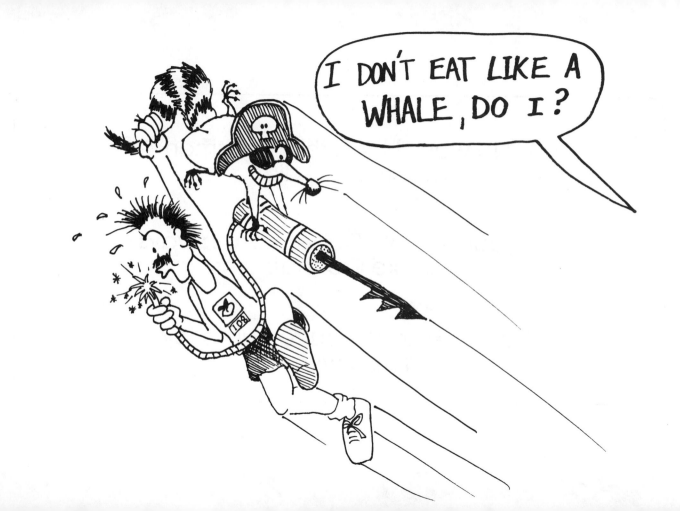

A. Gee, Honey, I don't think whales
can eat that much.

B. Impossible! Whales don't have hands
to shovel their food.

C. Don't be silly. You've hardly
touched your meal.

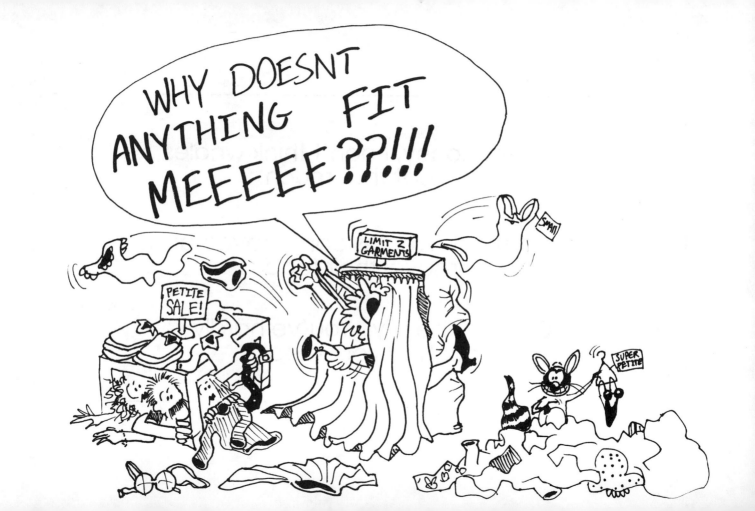

A. I take the fifth!

B. It's my fault—I must have shrunk *your* clothes in the dryer.

C. I love how everything hugs your curves.

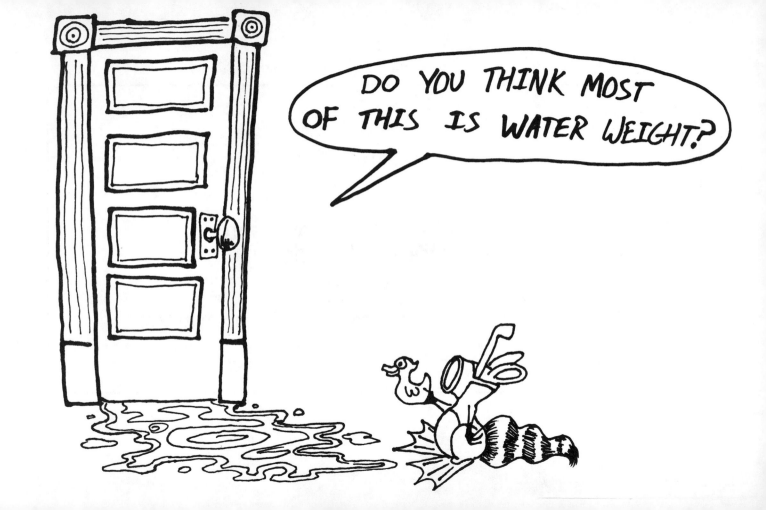

A. Yes, Darling. Your body uses water
to protect the baby.

B. Hey, when your water breaks,
this kid is going to ski out!

C. Could be – In Holland they just named
a dyke after you.

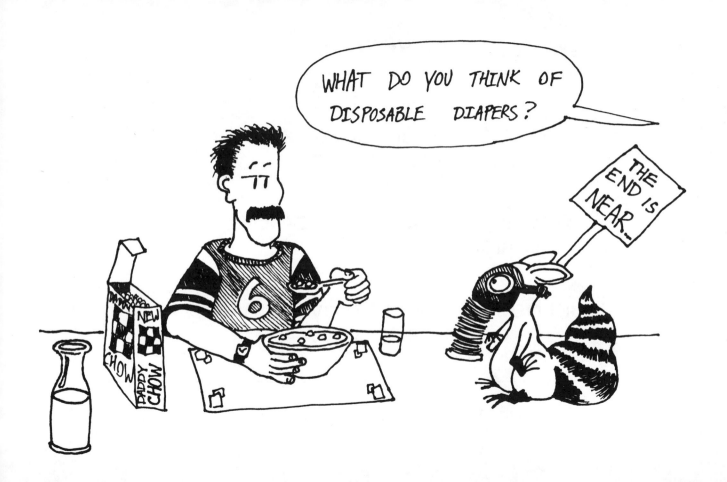

9.

A. Of course! Who wants to keep them?

B. I read that some of them hold up to 24 lbs!

C. They're disastrous to our environment.
Let's use a service – it's healthier and cheaper.

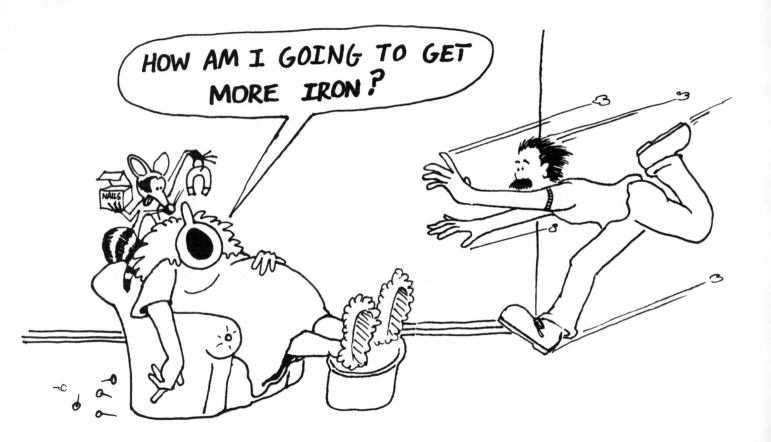

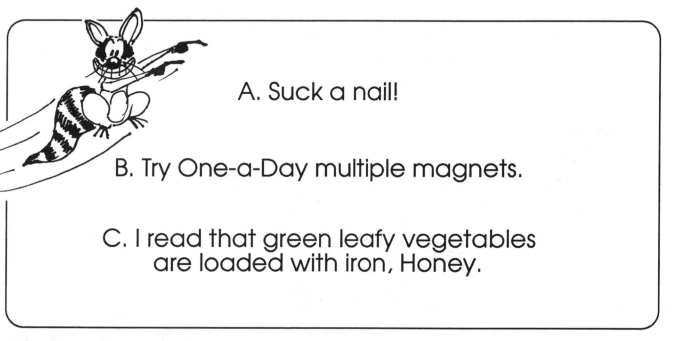

A. Suck a nail!

B. Try One-a-Day multiple magnets.

C. I read that green leafy vegetables
are loaded with iron, Honey.

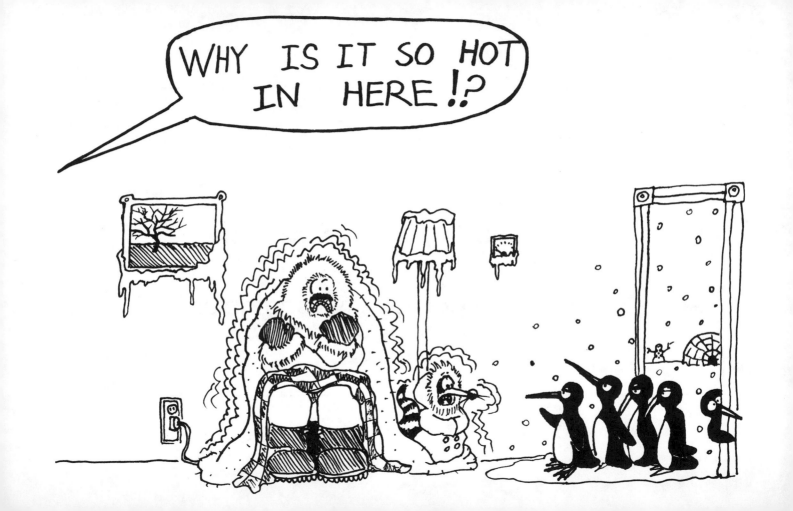

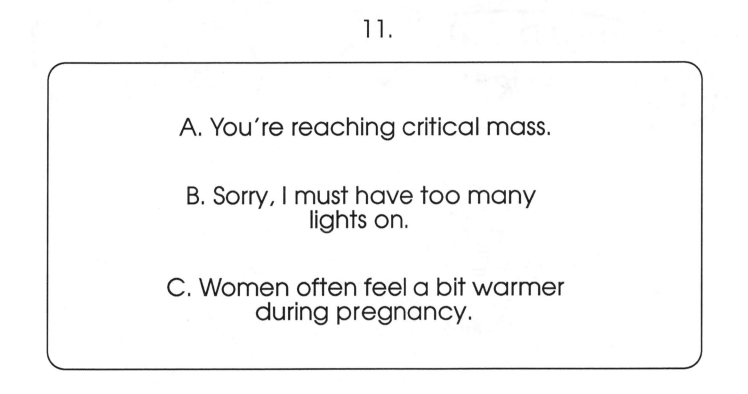

A. You're reaching critical mass.

B. Sorry, I must have too many
lights on.

C. Women often feel a bit warmer
during pregnancy.

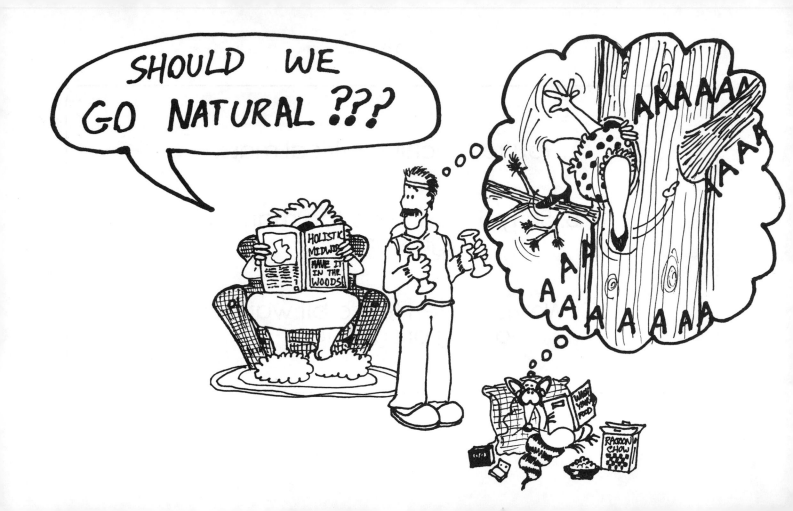

A. You mean like digging a hole
under the porch?

B. Sure beats unnatural.

C. From everything I've read,
it does give the baby the best start in life.

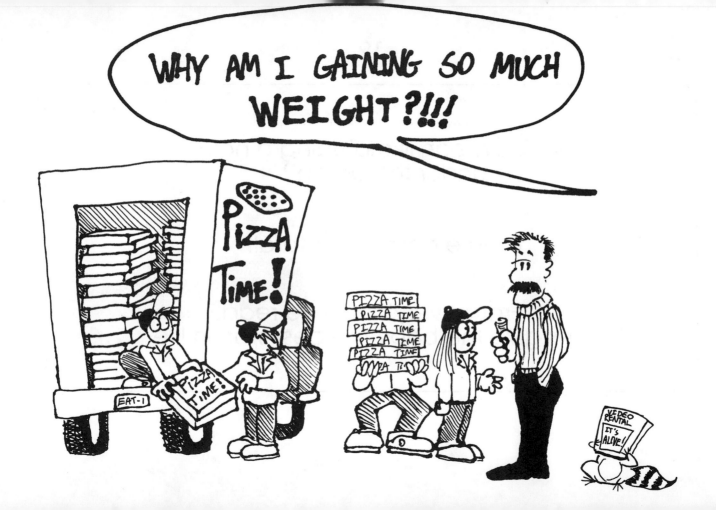

13.

A. Beats me – ask Pizza Hut.

B. Maybe it's something in the water.

C. It's your imagination.
You look incredible to me.

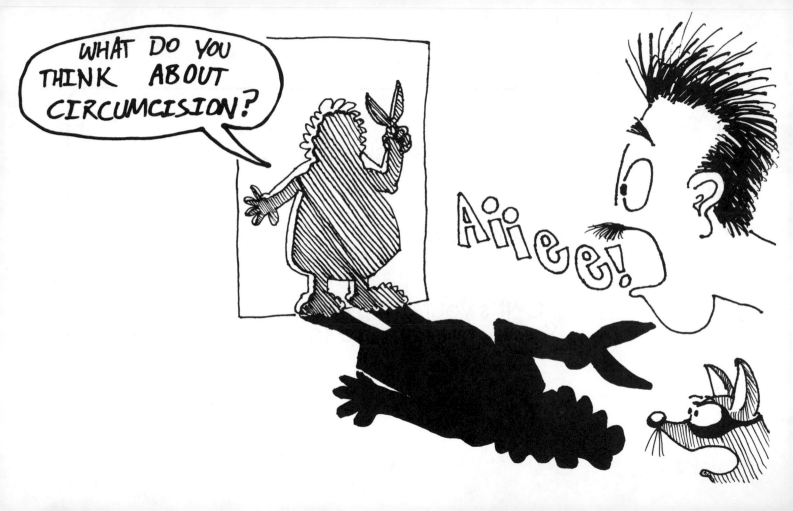

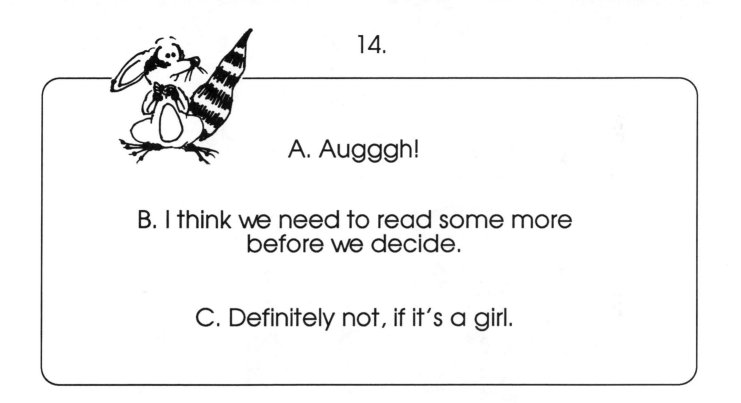

A. Augggh!

B. I think we need to read some more before we decide.

C. Definitely not, if it's a girl.

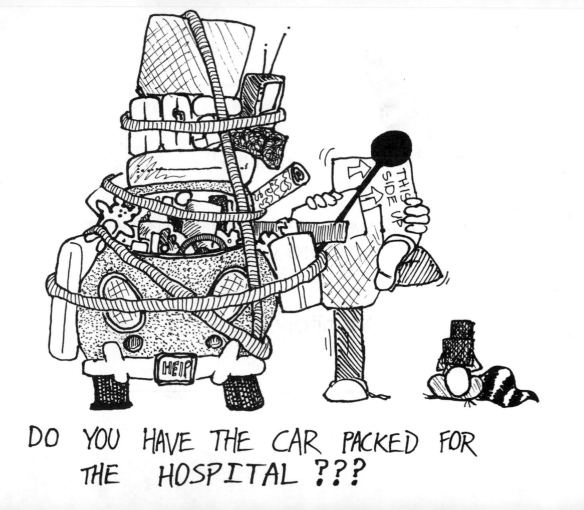

DO YOU HAVE THE CAR PACKED FOR
THE HOSPITAL ???

15.

A. No, I thought I'd wait until the end
of your second month.

B. Just relax, Darling,
I've taken care of everything.

C. Yes, Honeydrop, and there's even
some room for the baby.

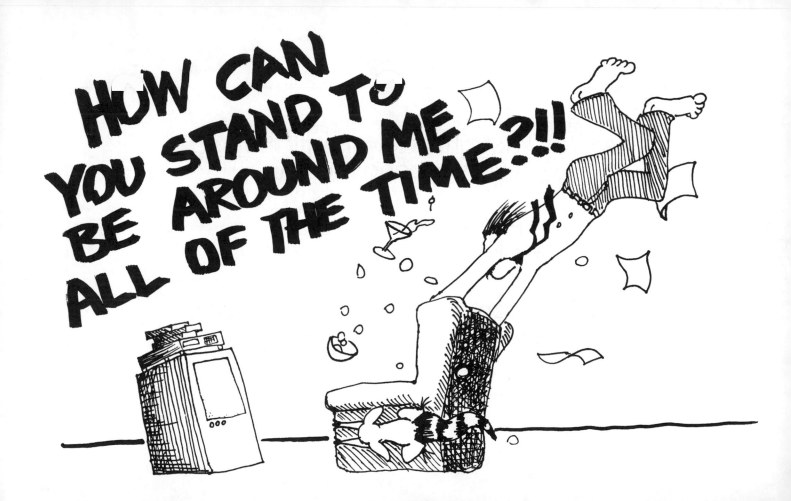

16.

A. My car's in the shop.

B. I've got medication.

C. I can't stand to be without you.

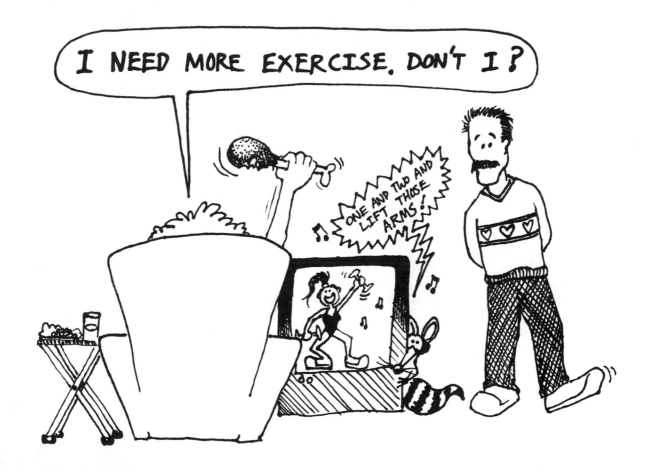

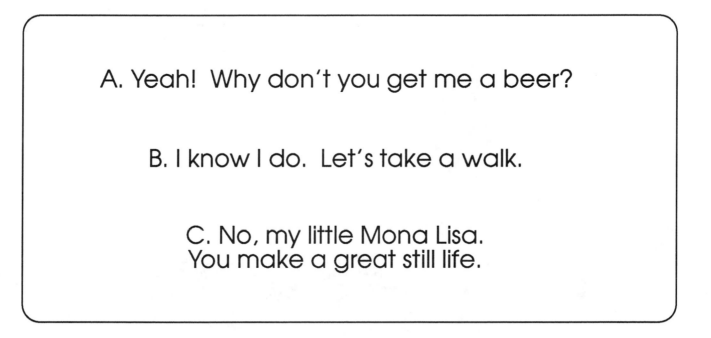

A. Yeah! Why don't you get me a beer?

B. I know I do. Let's take a walk.

C. No, my little Mona Lisa.
You make a great still life.

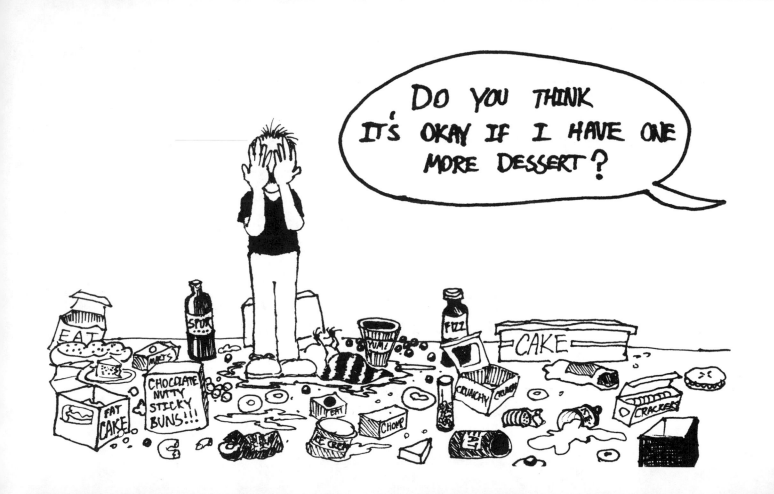

18.

A. Go for it! One more will break
the Guinness record.

B. Of course, cupcake, they're
cheaper by the cart!

C. You're already the sweetest thing
I've ever seen.

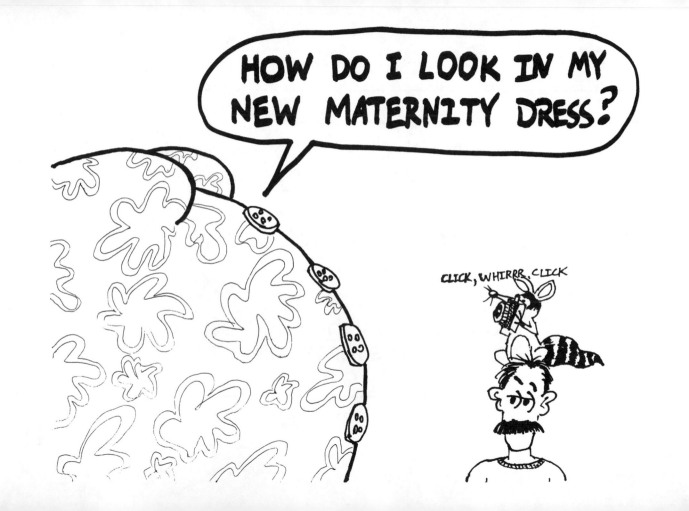

A. Next time I dream about you,
wear that dress.

B. Dress? I thought it was the
infield tarp for Yankee Stadium.

C. It's perfect, Love, and later it'll make
a great tent for the scout troop.

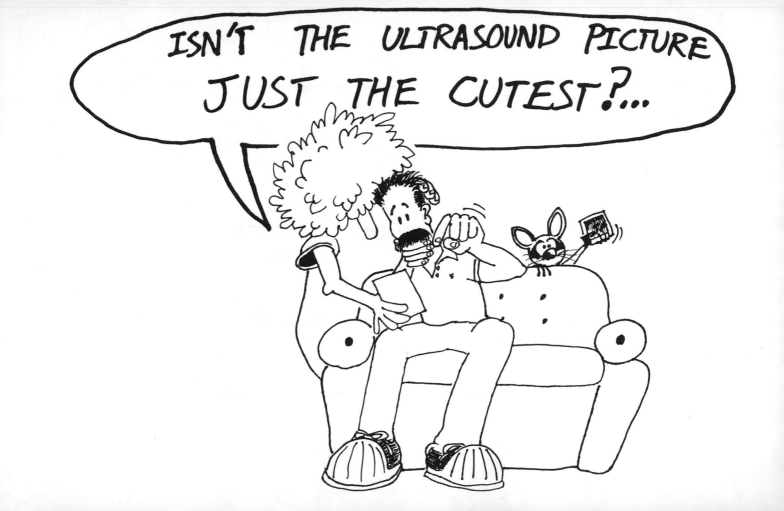

A. You're holding it upside down.

B. He's the cutest thing I've ever seen.

C. I think it looks like the Shroud of Turin!

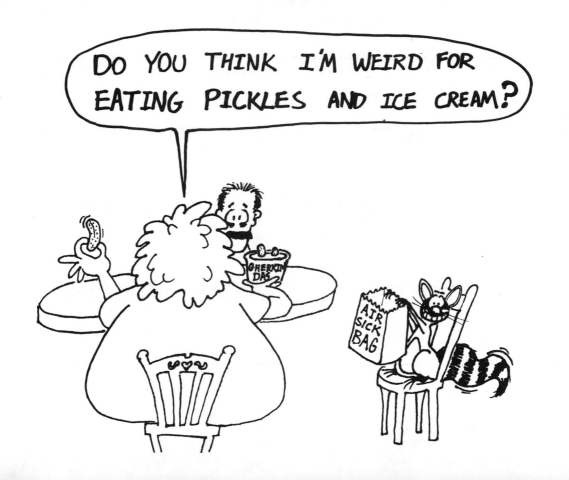

A. No, my sweet Gherkin, I think
I'm weird for watching you.

B. Are you kidding?
That's a great breakfast!

C. You're not weird. I'm sure your body
is craving this for a reason.

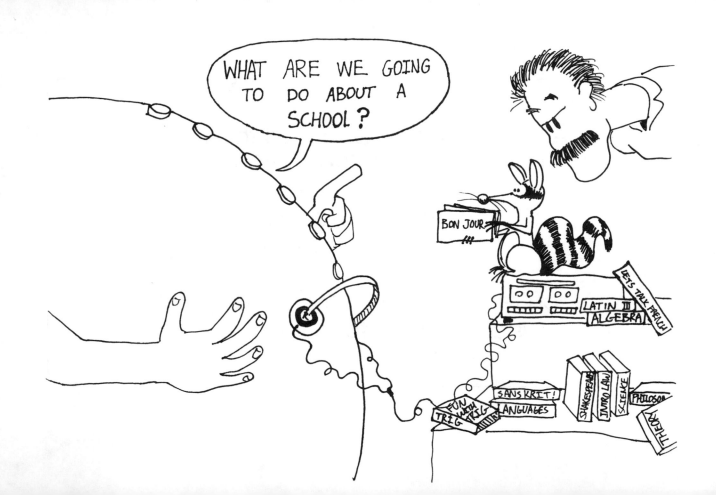

A. I called Harvard yesterday.
They want to see some grades first.

B. When the time comes, we'll find the
best school for our baby.

C. I think he should learn how to
drool first.

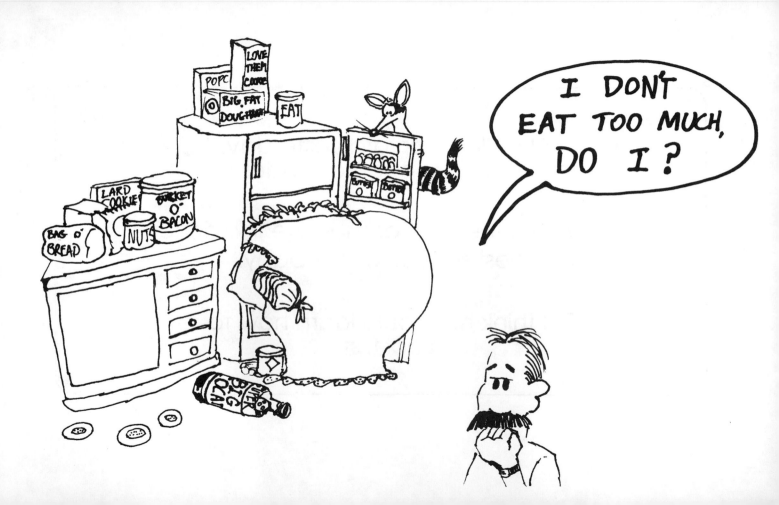

A. No, Honeybun, not for a small country.

B. Remember that you're making
our baby from what you're eating.
Sugar and spice is not everything nice.

C. No, Love Muffin. Now where do you want
these tubs of fudge ripple?

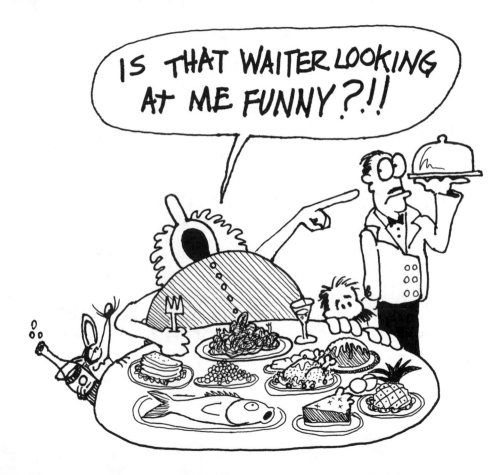

A. No, it's just your imagination. Now finish your
chocolate-covered shrimp and let's go.

B. No, Snookums, he's just never seen anyone
kill the entire buffet before!

C. He probably thinks you're some
movie star.

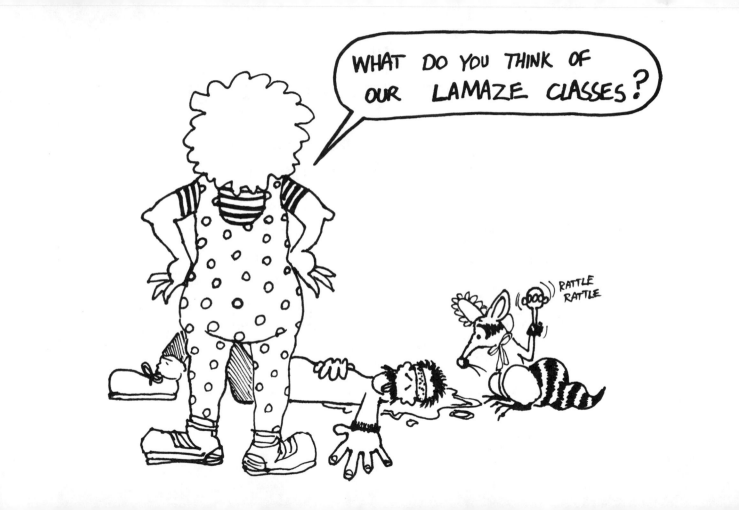

A. I'd rather take LeMans classes
where I drive you to the hospital and
drop you off.

B. I think birth classes are great.
Let's investigate to see
which is best for us.

C. All that panting and heavy breathing
reminds me of when you *got* pregnant!

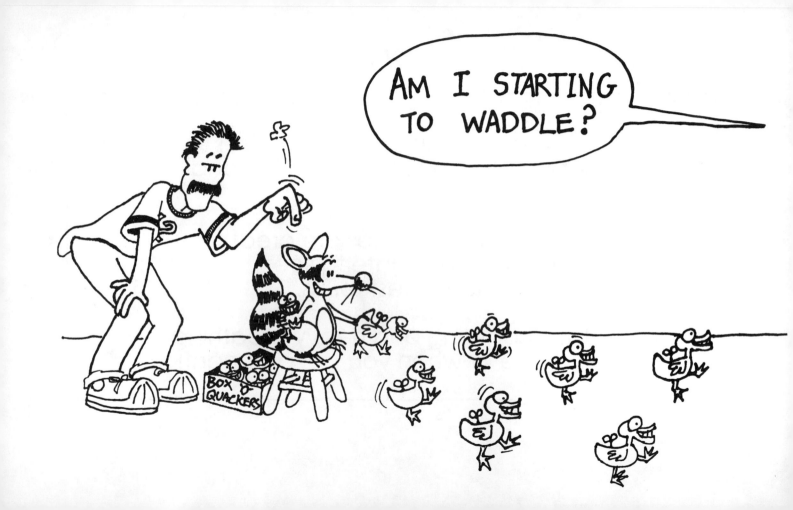

26

A. What did you say, Daffy?

B. No, Honey, but it might be safer
to stay in. It's hunting season.

C. Hey, Gorgeous, I was just going to say
what a sexy walk you have.

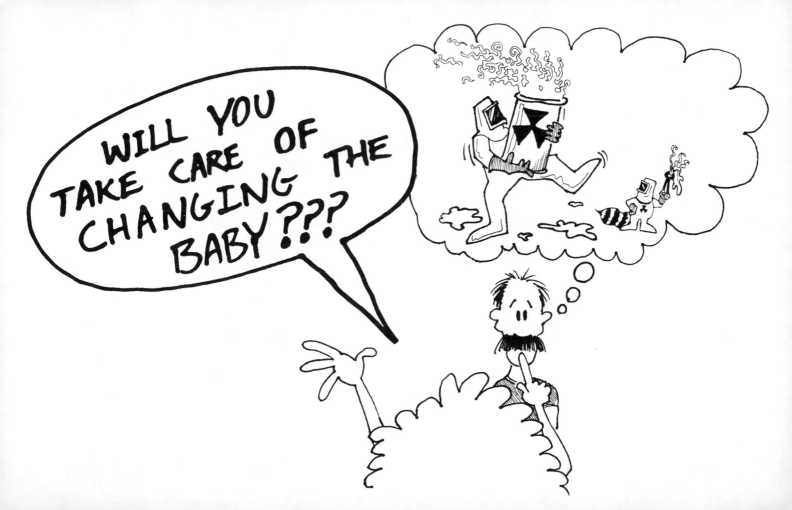

A. Changing it into what?

B. Sure, but that's going to be one
funky diaper by the time I get off work!

C. I'll be happy to help.

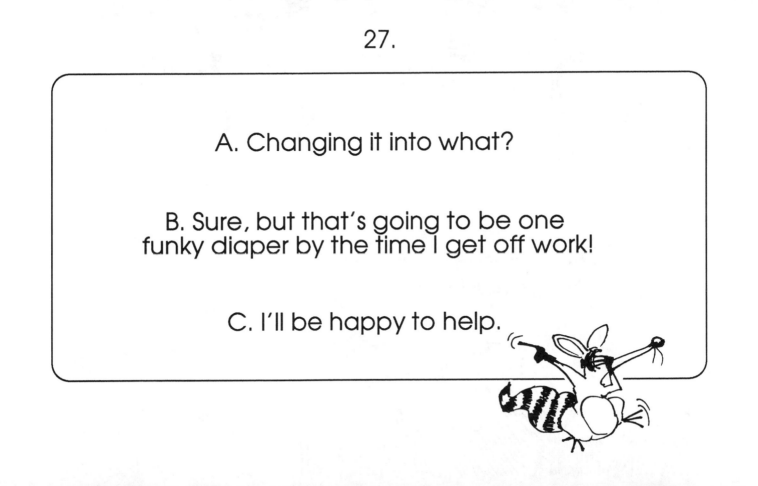

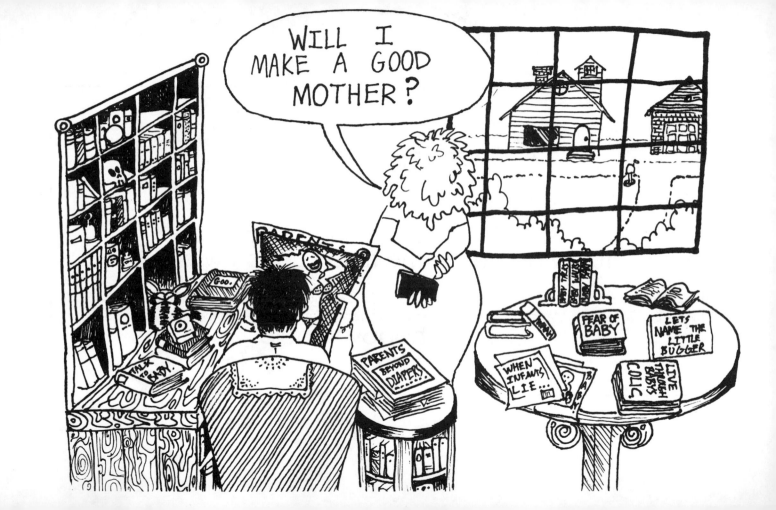

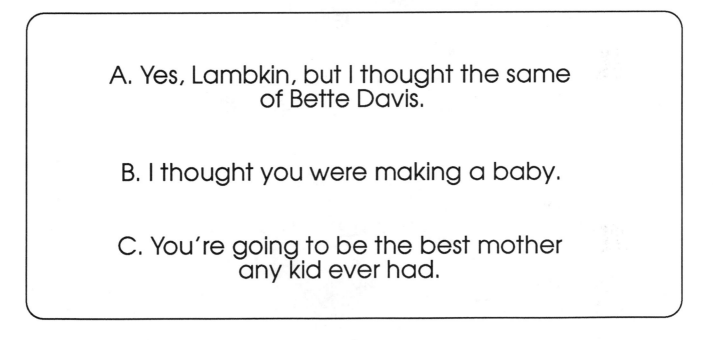

28

A. Yes, Lambkin, but I thought the same
of Bette Davis.

B. I thought you were making a baby.

C. You're going to be the best mother
any kid ever had.

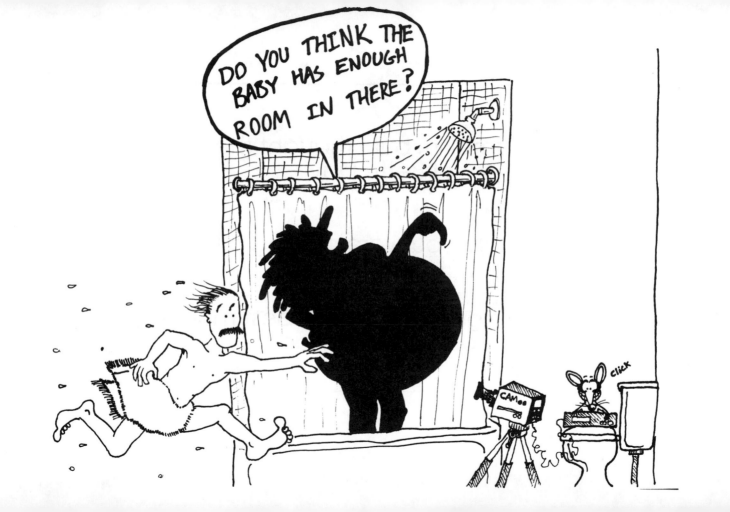

A. Don't worry – your body will adjust to give him all the room he needs.

B. He's got enough room to bowl!

C. Looks like he has plenty of "womb" to me.

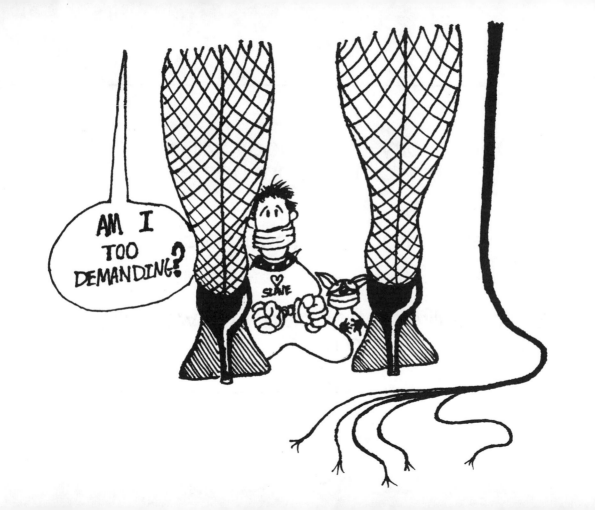

30

A. I don't think so, but the hostages are complaining.

B. If anything, you're *too* nice.

C. No, Honey, I enjoy scrubbing the floor with a toothbrush.

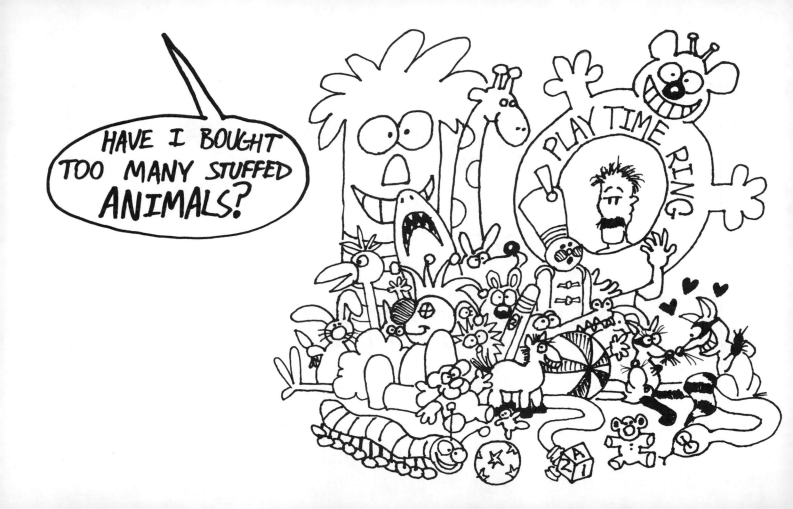

A. Not if we lived on the Ark!

B. No, Darling, but I think we need to save
some room for the baby.

C. No problem. I can always get
a second job.

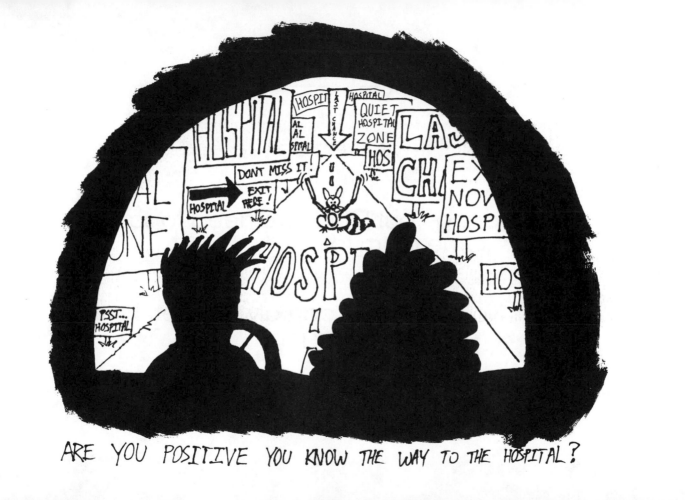

ARE YOU POSITIVE YOU KNOW THE WAY TO THE HOSPITAL?

32

A. Don't worry, Pumpkin.
Last visit, I left a trail.

B. I'll just follow the directions
you tattooed on my chest!

C. I have a map and the phone number
in the car, just in case.

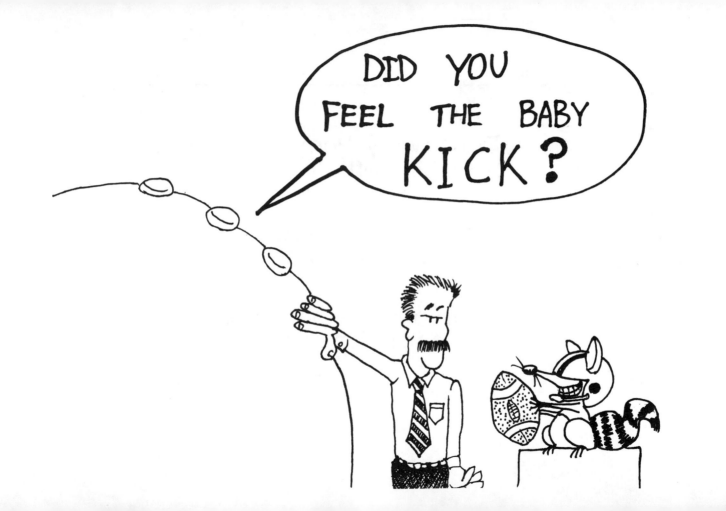

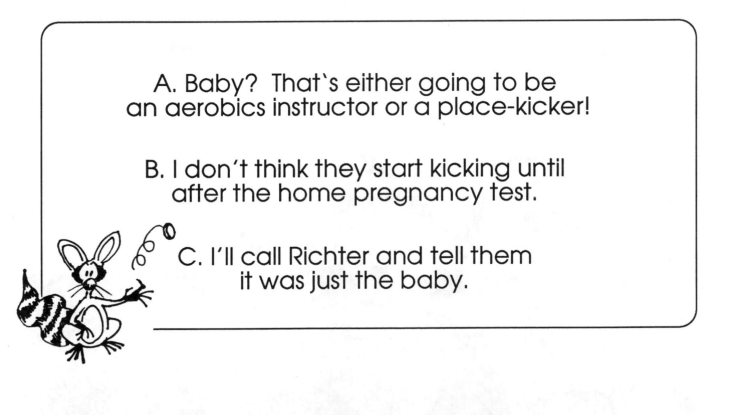

33

A. Baby? That's either going to be an aerobics instructor or a place-kicker!

B. I don't think they start kicking until after the home pregnancy test.

C. I'll call Richter and tell them it was just the baby.

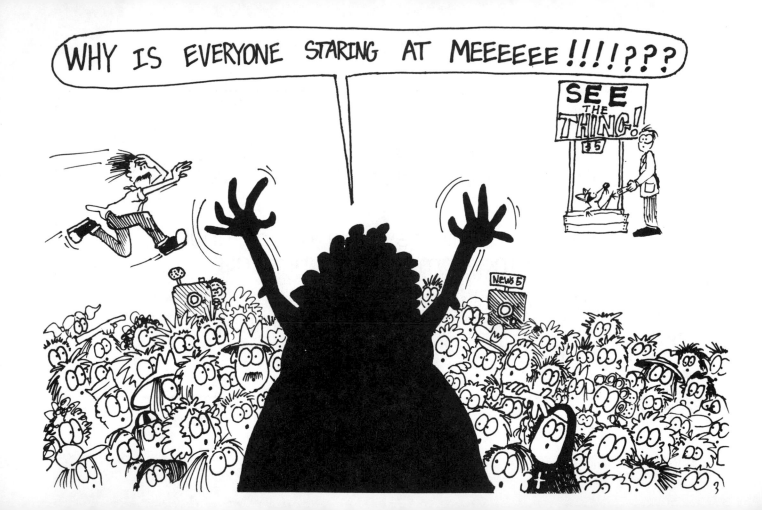

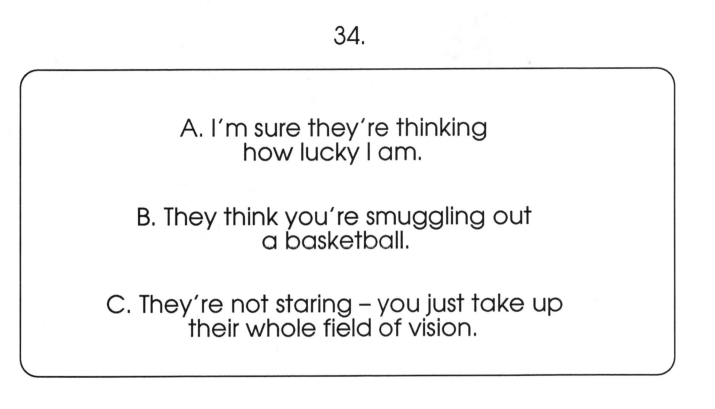

34

A. I'm sure they're thinking
how lucky I am.

B. They think you're smuggling out
a basketball.

C. They're not staring – you just take up
their whole field of vision.

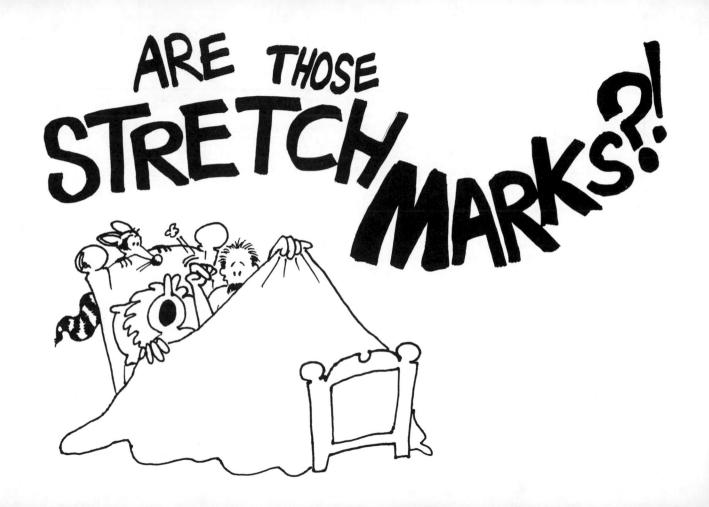

A. You mean that's not the road map
to the hospital?

B. I don't know what you're talking about.
I can't see anything.

C. You must have slept on a waffle iron.

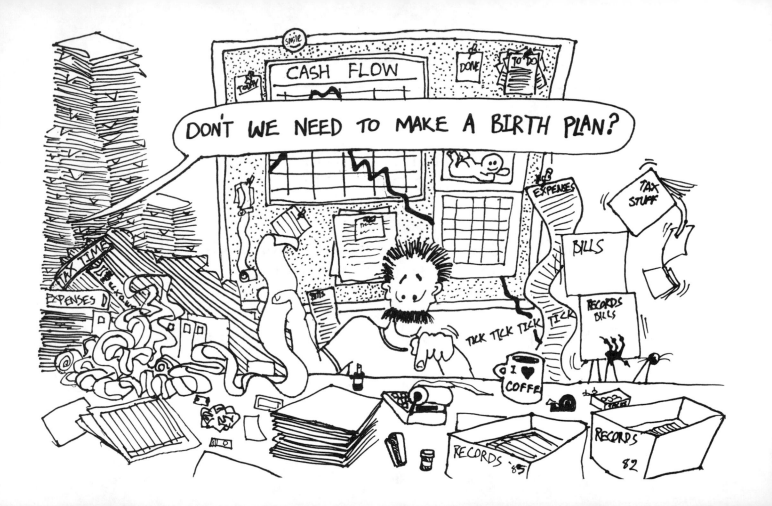

36

A. No, we need a payment plan.

B. Who needs a plan?
You push and I'll catch!

C. Yes, we do, but
let's leave room for flexibility.

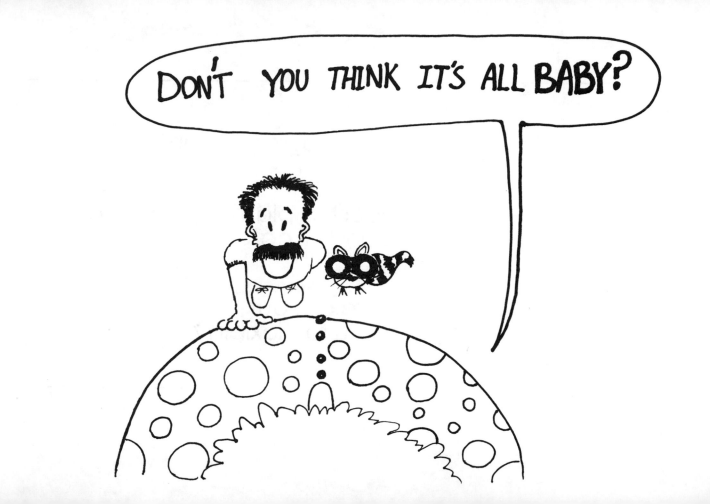

A. Sure, if the baby is King Kong.

B. All I know is it's all beautiful.

C. Certainly. Fifty-pound babies
are very common.

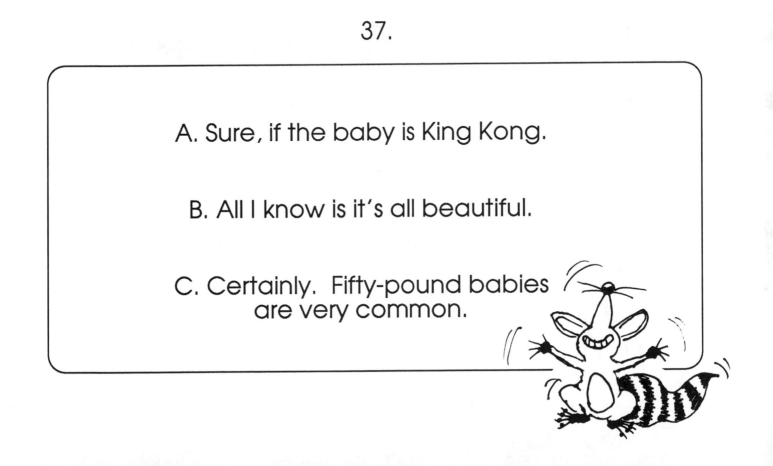

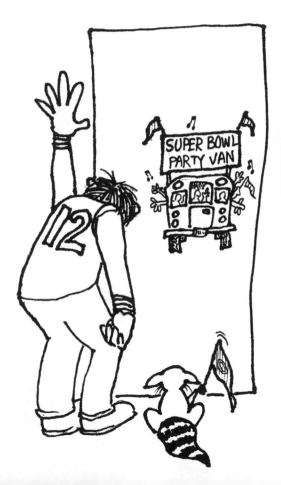
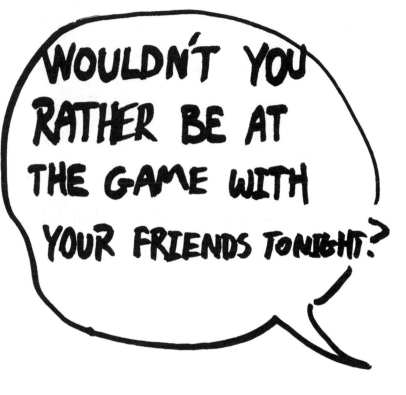

38

A. And miss the baby shower?
Are you kidding?

B. I treasure every minute we're together.

C. What's a couple of free box seats on the
fifty-yard line? There'll be other Super Bowls.

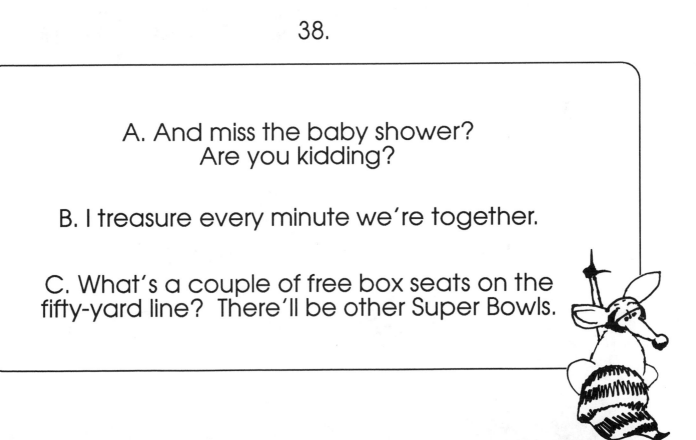

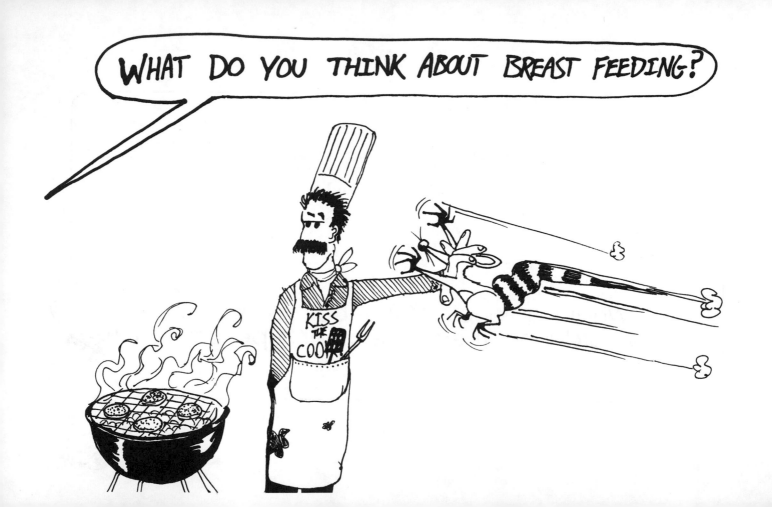

39

A. Taste great! Less filling!

B. Sure, if the baby will share.

C. I can't think of a heathier way
to start life.

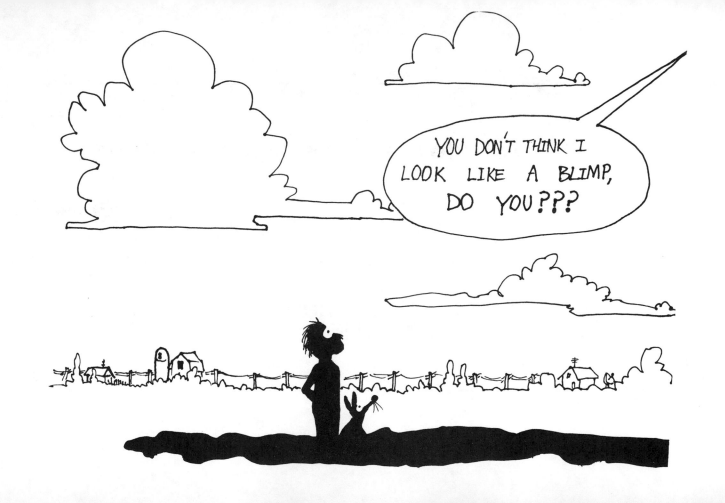

A. Stop kidding, Dumpling.
Blimps don't talk.

B. Now what? Did Goodyear call again?

C. You are blossoming like a beautiful
delicate rose.

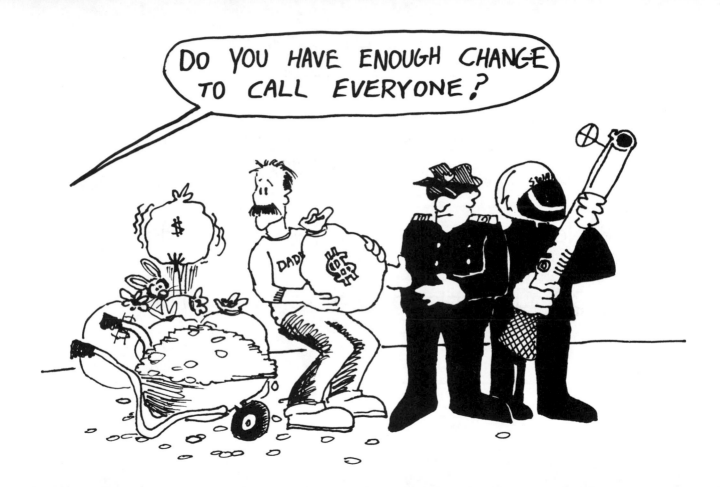

41.

A. I have enough change
to call everyone in Guam!

B. The Brinks truck is going
to meet us there.

C. I put an extra roll of quarters in the
suitcase next to the phone list.

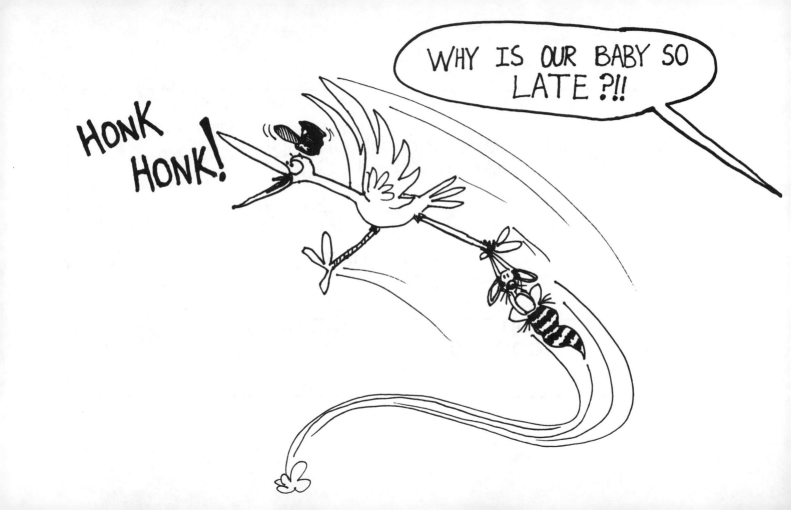

42

A. I'm sure she loves you so much
she doesn't want to leave.

B. Babies are always late. That's why
they can't keep a decent job.

C. Maybe she has a bad sense of direction.

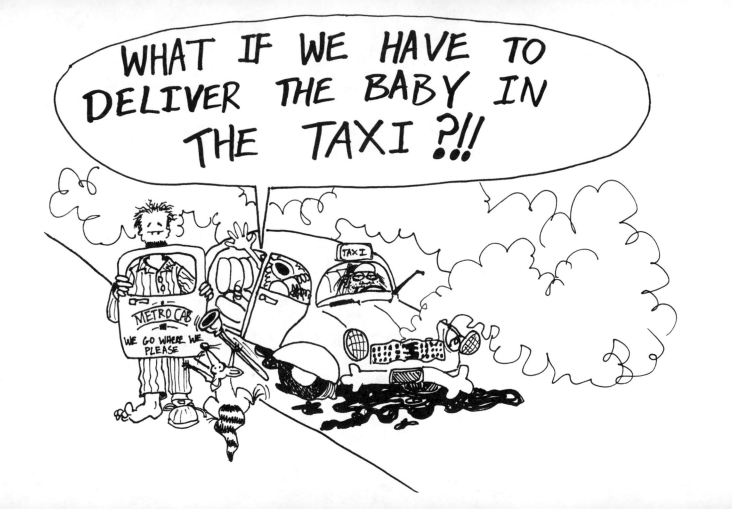

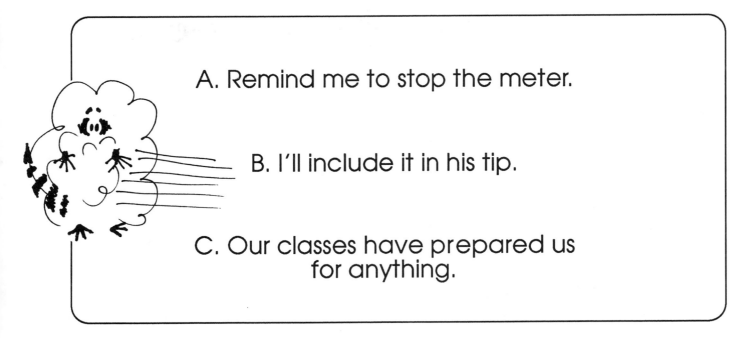

43

A. Remind me to stop the meter.

B. I'll include it in his tip.

C. Our classes have prepared us
for anything.

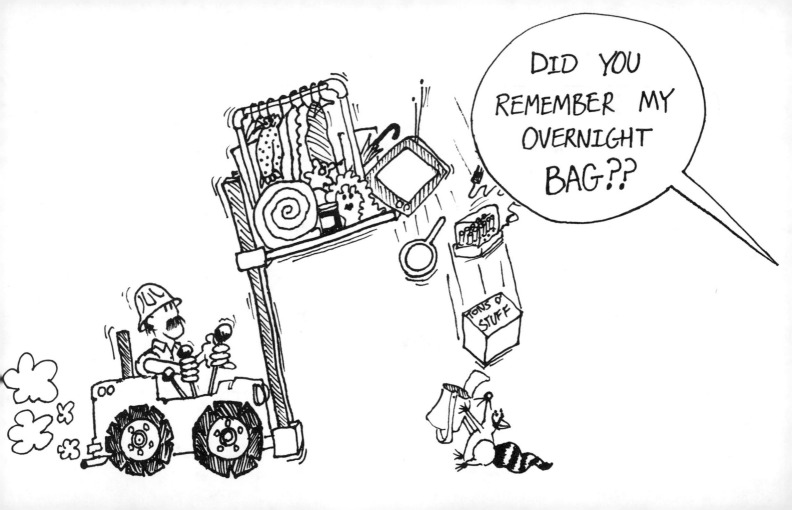

A. I remember where I left it.

B. We drove here in it!

C. I've brought everything we need,
my little Turtle Dove.

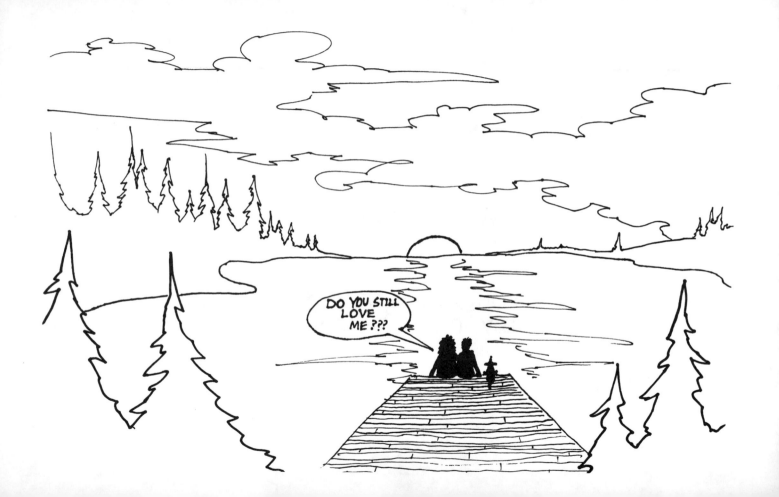

45

A. I'm amazed at how much more
I love you everyday.

B. Like the flowers love the spring.

C. My love grows for you with
each beat of my heart.

SCORING

1. C	10. C	19. A	28. C	37. B
2. B	11. C	20. B	29. A	38. B
3. A	12. C	21. C	30. B	39. C
4. B	13. C	22. B	31. B	40. C
5. C	14. B	23. B	32. C	41. C
6. C	15. B	24. C	33. C	42. A
7. C	16. C	25. B	34. A	43. C
8. A	17. B	26. C	35. B	44. C
9. C	18. C	27. C	36. C	45. C

Give yourself two points for every correct answer and one for every wrong answer.

If you scored **90,** congratulate yourself. You are the perfect Pregnant Husband.

If you scored between **89** and **80,** you're in for a long nine months.

If you scored between **79** and **70,** practice ducking.

If you scored between **69** and **60,** maybe you should have yourself sterilized.

If you scored between **59** and **50,** your wife has probably already done it for you.

If you scored below **50,** you should learn how to spell A-L-I-M-O-N-Y.

And After The Baby Comes

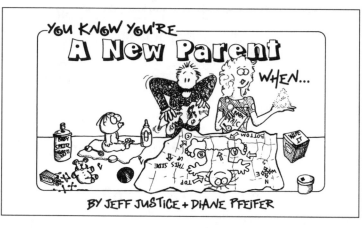

A hilarious look at those unforgettable moments when a new baby arrives. . . and stays!
The perfect gift for parents of newborns to toddlers.
Cartoons by Clark Taylor.

To order *The Pregnant Husband's Handbook* or *You Know You're A New Parent When*
by charge, call 1-800-875-7242 during business hours (EST)
or send check or money order for $5.95 plus $1 shipping to:

Strawberry Patch, Box 52404-Y, Atlanta, GA 30355